GRIFFONIA

A PREMIERE SOURCE OF 5-HYDROXYTRYPTOPHAN

Lane Williams

WOODLAND PUBLISHING
Pleasant Grove, UT

© 1998
Woodland Publishing
P.O. Box 160
Pleasant Grove, UT
84062

The information in this book is for educational purposes only and is not recommended as a means of diagnosing or treating an illness. All matters concerning physical and mental health should be supervised by a health practitioner knowledgeable in treating that particular condition. Neither the publisher nor author directly or indirectly dispense medical advice, nor do they prescribe any remedies or assume any responsibility for those who choose to treat themselves.

Table of Contents

Introduction 5
    Find a Natural Solution 7
Weight Management 7
Proteins and Amino Acids 10
Tryptophan 13
Serotonin 15
Serotonin and Obesity 18
5-Hydroxytryptophan 21
    5-HTP to Combat Depression 23
Griffonia simplicifolia 24
The Tryptophan Controversy 24
Some Final Thoughts about Obesity 28
Endnotes 29

GRIFFONIA

Introduction

Perhaps you have known someone like Phyllis, a 55-year-old housewife who was 45 pounds over her ideal weight. She exercised occasionally by taking walks. Sometimes, she started a diet.

She'd try to lose weight, but, instead, after a few weeks of success, became agitated and anxious, giving up the diet.

Phyllis, like some of your friends, started each day with a small breakfast, then ate a sensible lunch. But, by mid-afternoon, her mood usually went downhill. She became upset over trivial matters, and gradually, got bored, lonely and even depressed.

As evening set in, she began to eat, maybe bread or cheese followed by ice cream or cookies. Over the course of a day, she ate a healthy 2,100 calories at meal time, but 800 more came from snacking.

Or maybe you know someone like Laura, a 33-year-old administrator. She kept her calorie intake to a healthy 2,200 calories a day. She ate a well-balanced intake of food and exercised each day.

For seven days near the end of her monthly menstrual cycle she craved chocolate and ice cream. She couldn't quite understand why her balanced diet unraveled for these seven days. She ate starchy foods, and her calorie intake jumped by more than 40 percent to 3,000 calories a day. Her mood collapsed into anger, fatigue and anxiety. When she thought about losing weight, she figured a lack of self-control each month was part of the reason she was unsuccessful. It seemed that no matter how hard she tried, she couldn't keep away from a diet high in carbohydrates. She was successful in avoiding those calories only once, and her fatigue and sense of anxiousness only increased during those days of calorie-counting.

Both of these women became part of clinical trials for one of the first of the new generation of approved weight-loss drugs. The drug was dexfenfluramine, known more commonly by its brand name, Redux. Phyllis lost more than 11 pounds in three months. Laura found herself much more content during that difficult part of each month, and her carbohydrate cravings completely stopped.[1]

However, in September 1997, the United States Food and Drug Administration decided to ban the drug. At the same time, the agency also banned fenfluramine. (Together, this pair made up the famous phen-fen duo of diet drugs.)[2]

The scientific record lost track of what happened to Phyllis and Laura. Like many people, they may have begun to struggle again, watching the weight come back on, despite their best efforts at diet and exercise.

So what are your friends like Phyllis and Laura to do?

Find a Natural Solution

Though many companies and researchers are finding exciting ways to deal naturally with weight management problems, one natural solution that has emerged is clearly one of the most exciting. It is an herb known as *Griffonia simplicifolia*, a West African seed from a plant used commonly for food and medicine.

Griffonia is high in 5-hydroxytryptophan (5-HTP), a substance that can have the same effects as dexfenfluramine on appetite and weight control, but through a different, and evidently much safer, mechanism.[3]

But more on that later. First, let's talk more about the reality of weight management and the obsessions we have with it.

Weight Management

One of the great ironies and lessons of women like Phyllis and Laura is that the way we eat can be much more complicated than merely self-control. Laura did most things expected of her in that she exercised, ate a balanced diet and counted calories. Still, she was unable to control her weight and calorie intake for one week per month.

In many people, such a desire to control weight coupled with a seeming inability to control food intake can lead to guilt and shame. One of the great hopes of this new generation of natural solutions may be not just that weight management will improve, but shame will decrease as people come to understand that much of our binging is as natural a result of bodily cravings just as taking a long drink from a clear mountain spring is the result of thirst.

The shame of weight gain runs deep in Western culture. From as early as the 1700s, weight-loss gurus focused on body size, and their solution was to merely cut calories and food intake. One notable man, Sonorio Sonorio, invented a unique chair/scale. On one end of his pulley-like scale sat a chair in an open, phone booth-shaped container. Secured by a rope, the chair dangled just above the floor. A weight hung on the other end of the this rope/pulley system to keep the chair balanced only an inch or two above the floor. Sonorio sat in the chair as he ate. If he ate too much—too much as he reasoned anyway—his weight would increase, and the chair would touch the floor. This was his obsessive way of keeping his weight in check—merely keeping the chair dangling in midair.[4]

Sonorio's legacy is still with us. How many people like Phyllis and Laura focus on overeating as the sole cause of weight gain? For many years in fact, scientists supported the view that the only reason people gained weight was because they ate too much. Obese people, the reasoning went, were fat because they lacked self-control—because they were bad people, gluttons, if you will. Never mind that much concerning this philosophy is chicken fat and ready to be thrown aside with the moldy leftovers of yesteryear.

This philosophy of self-control became so ingrained in Western culture that by 1880 people paid money to see a man named Henry Tanner avoid food. After an 11-day fast, people began to pay 25 cents each for the privilege of watching him lose weight. This led to an entire generation of "hunger artists" who went on long fasts for profit. One, Giovanni Succi, fasted for 45 days as a way to make a living.[5]

Though many still hold to the gluttony view, science has found something wrong with this understanding of self-control, and its role in weight-management.

One of the most insightful bits of research came from devoted American men who avoided military service in World War II for religious reasons—the conscientious objectors. Rather than go and fight, these men contributed in another way to relieve suffering during that terrible time.

These conscientious objectors went on carefully supervised low-calorie diets—a kind of forced starvation—to help officials learn how to heal starving, concentration camp victims. At the University of Minnesota, scientists observed the precise intake of food these men ate as they came out of the imposed restrictions. These observations helped scientists predict what prisoners would do when they were liberated and thus helped caregivers improve the healing process.

As the objectors emerged from the diets, they grew increasingly hungry over time and, in fact, weighed five percent more on average when they ended the study than when they began it.[6]

In the same way, starving refugees after World War I and famished prisoners after World War II tended to weigh more after they gained the weight back than before their ordeals began.[7] These examples show that hunger and weight loss are more complex than merely self-control. Weight management involves a wide variety of bodily systems, many of which are only now emerging into scientific view.

Meal portions tend to be too large in North American meals, and much can be said for eating less as a matter of habit, but these examples prove long-term weight-management is more complicated than merely sitting in a chair hanging an inch or two above the ground.

For men and women like Phyllis and Laura, their desire for snacks high in carbohydrates and the depression that often accompanies their cravings comes not so much from losing "self-control" or from feeling guilty, but rather from an in-born desire to meet the body's real needs. As we'll discuss later, many of these cravings are physical effects of nutritional problems as real as hunger pains after a 24-hour fast or as natural as dry thirst on a desert island.

Yet people on a desert island don't feel guilty for feeling thirsty, while many feel guilty for their desires to eat certain snack foods. Should they feel guilty? No.

Of course, taking a drink from a mountain stream is the best solution for thirst, but eating snacks really isn't the best long-term solution to these cravings because many of these foods can lead to obesity and poorer overall health. Of course, we're still advocating that people avoid many of those unhealthy snack foods, but rather than cut through the depression and anxiety to avoid those foods, what people need to do is find new solutions in their diet.

The 5-HTP in griffonia is one of those emerging solutions. Within the body, 5-HTP changes to serotonin, one of the most important natural transmitters in our nerves. Essentially, when we're low on serotonin, we feel cravings and depression. So, if you can influence the body's use of serotonin, you can influence the body's appetite and mood.

First, however, to understand serotonin and its role in our diet, we must understand more clearly the natural world it comes from. That means understanding a little more about the microscopic world of proteins and amino acids.

Proteins and Amino Acids

The ancient Greeks, as well as many ancient cultures, wondered what food really was. That is, if you were to break food down to its most basic elements, what would finally result?

Is there one kind of food? Or are there several? Hippocrates said, "There is but one food, but there exist several forms of food." He believed that variety existed in food, but, at their essence they were one.

Similarly, the great Roman physician Galen thought that food was one basic nutrient, and during digestion food could be broken down. Though far from the truth, this view remained the dominant view for centuries. The truth, of course, is that food contains a wide variety of elements, each with unique functions. Food is fat, carbohydrates, minerals, vitamins, phytochemicals . . . and protein.

In the early 18th century, Italian scientist Iacopo Bartolomeo Beccari ground wheat up into a fine flour and then soaked the flour in water. He found that he could make a starch and a liquid gluten from soaking the flour. The starch would ferment the way vegetables do, but the gluten would begin to stink and rot, much like meat does. This was an important beginning inprotein science.[8]

This kind of division became the way carbohydrates and proteins were distinguished. Carbohydrates were vegetable-like, and proteins were meat-like.

Protein, for many years, was seen as the central, only vital nutrient, in keeping with the tradition of Galen and Hippocrates. Indeed, the word *protein* comes from the Greek word meaning primary.

An important shift in thinking was a result of the French scientist Antoine Lavoisier, who observed that life is a chemical function. (Lavoisier was controversial enough to lose his life during the French Revolution.)[9]

Proteins were first recognized as unique entities in the 1830s by Gerardus Mulder.[10] By 1902, Emil Fisher established the general structure of protein.

Indeed, proteins are large molecules that stretch to hundreds of atoms. About 20 common amino acids, still smaller molecules, combine in numerous fashions to make proteins. Other more rare amino acids and other chemicals, such as minerals and vitamin-like compounds, combine to make still other proteins. Some proteins may contain 100 amino acids.

Some proteins build cellular structure while others complete vital human functions. These vital proteins include enzymes, which help the body produce chemical reactions and build cells; hemoglobin, an important component of our blood; hormones, which help cells communicate with each other; and antibodies, which help the body fight off infection. Other common proteins include collagen and keratin, which support body tissues and gives them strength.

A simple bacterium can produce between 2,000 and 4,000 different proteins for its use. The human body produces as many as 50,000 different proteins. Each protein is a three-dimensional structure, and the unique shape of a protein determines its specific function.

At the heart of each cell is our DNA—the deoxyribonucleic acid. The DNA helps cells produce proteins.[11]

Part of good nutrition means getting the right amino acids through a well balanced diet. Twelve of the 20 vital amino acids are produced within the body; however, eight of the amino acids must come from diet and nutrition.

These eight amino acids that must come from diet and nutrition are the essential amino acids. Without them, we suffer the gradual effects of starvation where our bodies consume their own muscle to survive, the belly swells and death results.

These eight essential amino acids are as vital to nutrition as vitamin C or iron. The eight essential amino acids are

- Isoleucine
- Leucine
- Lysine
- Methionine

- Phenylalanine
- Threonine
- Valine
- Tryptophan.[12]

As for the basic structure, amino acids have three main portions. First, a group of atoms—one nitrogen and two hydrogens—sit on one side of the molecule. The second portion includes one carbon, two oxygens and one hydrogen. These two groups naturally connect, sort of like magnets, based on their natural electrical charge. This creates the string of amino acids leading to the formation of protein.

The third part of each amino acid is different for each and accordingly gives each a unique function.[13]

The least common of these eight essential amino acids is tryptophan, yet science has found a remarkable number of functions and effects that emerge from tryptophan. It is the effects of tryptophan, and specifically, the effects of tryptophan's relatives like 5-HTP and serotonin that give griffonia its excitement and emerging power in the natural community.

Tryptophan

Around 1889, Sir Frederick Gowland Hopkins became fascinated with a simple question: What makes the wings of some butterflies yellow?

During his research in 1902, Hopkins indentified the amino acid and named it tryptophan.[14]

The isolation of tryptophan came following years of research where biochemists would test various proteins with chemicals and see what colors resulted. Tryptophan caused a red pigment to emerge.

Typtophan is less common than many of the other essential amino acids, and indeed, several studies indicate that people need less tryptophan than, for example, valine. In fact, science shows that humans need about four times as much valine as tryptophan to survive.[15]

However, tryptophan regulates many of the basic human processes. Bodily processes change the chemical structure of tryptophan and convert it into serotonin, which helps the body send messages in the brain and along nerves; melatonin, helps regulate sleep; picolinate, helps metals, particularly zinc, transport into cells; and kynurenine. It is also a precursor to the B vitamin niacin.

An average daily diet contains about 500 to 1,000 mg of tryptophan. Animal proteins contain about 1.4 percent tryptophan and vegetable proteins about 1 percent.[16]

In nature, soybeans and soy products are the highest natural sources of tryptophan.[17] Cereal grains and many seeds, such as sesame seeds, are notable vegetable sources as well.[18]

Some research has shown that tryptophan may be vital in the way certain proteins, such as the human growth hormone, do their jobs in the body.[19]

Most tryptophan research is a fairly recent phenomenon. Nearly a quarter of a century ago, a group of interested scientists met in Italy to discuss their research on this important biochemical. Though the group expressed excitement at being able to meet together as colleagues, many longtime experts figured there wasn't enough direction of study on tryptophan to justify another meeting three years hence.

These experts were wrong. Rather than fading from focus in research, tryptophan scholarship has emerged as one of the most important biological achievements of the twentieth century.[20]

The conference has continued to meet every three years since. Scientists compare notes on this fertile area of study. In the most recent meeting—summer 1995—scientists from around the world delivered nearly 120 separate lectures and papers on tryptophan and its family of related chemicals.

There's research about melatonin, which helps to regulate sleep and is a byproduct of tryptophan. There's also research on kyurenine and quinolinic acid, other derivatives of tryptophan and their relationship to pain, inflammation and cell damage.

Most remarkable of all, perhaps, is the research on serotonin.

Serotonin

For each breath we take, each thought we have, each muscle we twitch, our remarkable, unusual nerve cells send electric and chemical signals throughout our complex nervous system. Serontonin's role in this process is vital.

Most cells are round, much like a fried egg, with a nucleus—the yolk, so to speak—in the middle of a broader cell enclosed in roundish, fatty walls.

Nerve cells, called neurons, however, send long, octupus-like arms reaching out from the center of the nerve cell toward their nearest neighbors. Our brain is a collection of neurons.

These arms reach for a handshake, if you will, with neighboring neurons, but never quite reach. Each neuron is separated from its neighbor by an ever-so-narrow gap. Still, if there were no way for the brain's message to jump this barrier, then the narrow gap might as well be the Grand Canyon.

Serotonin, one of the most important neurotransmitters, acts as the bridge from one neuron to the next. It acts as a courier that helps pass along the brain's command to the lungs to take a breath and that relays the finger's message that a pan is hot.

Without serotonin, as you might imagine, we would die.

With little surprise, you can find, then, numerous reasons why serotonin, called 5-hydroxytryptamine, is playing a primary part in the most recent research about tryptophan. You can understand why scientists have continued to gather information in this area of study for a quarter of a century.

Consider a few of serotonin's effects:

- In experiments dating back to the mid 1960s, scientists observed that if you deplete serotonin in the brain, the chances increase that an epileptic will suffer a seizure. Similarly, researchers find less tryptophan in the blood of epileptics than in those who don't suffer from the disease.[21]
- Some early research with serotonin also shows that it can have an anticonvulsive effect.[22]
- Serotonin may decrease our perception of pain—at least some kinds of pain. For about a decade, scientists studying serotonin have observed that as serotonin levels rise in the central nervous system, the pain threshold rises, making our perception of pain less, especially for lower back pain.

  This area of research is only beginning, and much needs to be done to better understand serotonin. The promise of long-term relief from pain still remains one of medicine's important quests, and serotonin-related therapies may be an important part of this quest.[23]

  Another part of the this research shows that morphine produces more serotonin than the body has normally, and, similarly, short-term stress can release serotonin, thereby causing some temporary pain relief.

  Another significant fact in pain research is that medical practitioners often give antidepressants—because

they cause more serotonin to be available in the nerves—as a medication among others to battle chronic pain.[24]
- Migraine sufferers clearly face problems when the amount of serotonin decreases in their bodies. Several tests have shown that drugs that decrease the amount of serotonin cause pain in migraine-sufferers.[25]
- Though much research remains to be done, strong evidence from scientific studies show that when scientists lower the amount of serotonin in the brain they also cause depression in their patients.

One interesting study at McGill University in Montreal fed subjects a diet known as acute tryptophan depletion. Basically, the researchers fed their test subjects a mixture of all the essential amino acids except tryptophan. This kind of feeding caused the body to manufacture proteins, and since the body needed tryptophan for those proteins, the body pulled tryptophan from the reserves already floating in the bloodstream or elsewhere in the body. Within five hours, the amount of tryptophan in the blood dropped by as much as 80 percent. Researchers have noted that in many cases, particularly in those people with a history of depression, a blue mood sets in. Scientists also deduced that serotonin in the brain is also reduced.

(Because there's no ethical way to do this kind of research for more than a few hours, it remains hard to determine what effect such tryptophan deprivation might cause over a long period of time. Indeed, most researchers only deplete tryptophan from the diet of their test subjects for no longer than five hours.)

Accordingly, it seems clear that serotonin does play some important role in mood, particularly depression.[26]

Similarly, in AIDS patients suffering with mental disorders and depression, it isn't uncommon to find the amount of tryptophan in their bloodstreams at only 60 percent of average.[27]

As is clear from this research, serotonin is a remarkable biochemical and plays an important role in a wide variety of disorders. According to University of Mississippi researcher Ronald F. Bore, serotonin is "The Neurotransmitter of the '90s." He writes that "of the chemical neurotransmitter substances . . . serotonin is perhaps the most implicated in the etiology or treatment of various disorders, particularly those of the central nervous system, including anxiety, depression, obsessive-compulsive disorder, schizophrenia, stroke, obesity, pain, hypertension, vascular disorders, migraine, and nausea."[28]

Serotonin and Obesity

The idea that serotonin might affect our appetite is less than a quarter of a century old,[29] but in that short time, a solid theory has emerged from numerous research projects dealing with serotonin research: When the brain, particularly the area known as the satiety center, has more serotonin available, then our feelings of satiety—the feeling of being full—increase.[30] And accordingly, we eat less.

One of the more interesting applications of this idea comes from research done on patients suffering from cancer, AIDS or a similar long-term disease. To doctors, one of the most significant challenges of treating these illnesses is that their patients often lose large amounts of weight, sometimes very quickly. The loss of weight makes the patient weak and thus hinders the effects of drugs designed to cure.

Therefore, doctors want patients to gain or at least maintain their weight. Some treatments of this disease-related weight-loss are designed to decrease the amount of serotonin between the nerves. These treatments have proven effective in helping the patients maintain weight.[31]

Of course, for people like Phyllis and Laura, the problem is exactly the opposite. They want to eat less; they want to lose weight.

In the modern United States, obesity is a silent killer. It is a factor in heart disease, some forms of cancer and diabetes. Tens of thousands of people die each year from obesity-related conditions.

Given the results of these studies, it seems that a reasonable approach to dealing with appetite would be to simply increase the amount of serotonin in the brain, thereby making us want to eat less.

Why not give people a shot? How about a pill that contains serotonin, perhaps flavored with orange? Unfortunately, the body doesn't work that way. To protect our brains from the number of strange chemicals we encounter, nature has provided a protection known as the blood-brain barrier. This barrier prevents plain serotonin from crossing from the bloodstream into the brain, just as it helps protect against dangerous chemicals from crossing into the brain.

So, we must work through other methods to increase the serotonin or its effectiveness in the body. For example, we could merely eat a diet high in tryptophan and let it change through 5-HTP to become serotonin.

Logic might suggest, therefore, that merely eating a diet high in protein—one high in meat, for example—would be useful in getting tryptophan into the system because tryptophan is part of protein. Similarly, logic might suggest that we wouldn't want to eat those potato chips, high in carbohydrates, which lack tryptophan.

Again, there's a problem with this logic. Meat and many high-protein diets are also high in the other essential amino acids. Tryptophan, indeed, makes up only about 1 percent of the overall protein content of foods, so there are more of the other amino acids in the diet.

Some of those essential amino acids, notably valine, leucine and isoleucine, compete with tryptophan to cross the blood-brain barrier. So, even though we may eat a lot of protein that includes tryptophan, the blood-brain barrier lets less tryptophan cross into the brain than other amino acids.

Therefore, though we may eat lots of protein, less serotonin in the brain will emerge, and we will begin that carbohydrate thirst Laura and Phyllis complained about.

Carbohydrates do not contain tryptophan. What gives? Why would our bodies want carbohydrates?

Many carbohydrates help the body release insulin, which not only regulates the sweet sugar in our diet but also helps improve the ratio of tryptophan to these other amino acids in the blood. That is, when we eat carbohydrates, we make tryptophan, and therefore serotonin is able cross the blood-brain barrier more readily because there are fewer competing amino acids seeking to cross into the brain at the same gate.[32]

So these carbohydrates, ultimately, lead to a short-lived release of serotonin in the brain. We feel better. You've probably noticed how a fresh bag of potato chips can make you feel better, seemingly, from the first bite.

Of course, one of the problems with the carbohydrates we eat is that they often take the form of snack foods, rich in unhealthy fats and other ingredients that put on the weight or hinder our healthy lifestyles.

This set of facts seem to argue in favor, incidentally, of beginning each day with a healthy breakfast rich in whole grains, which have some tryptophan, but are high in carbohydrates. Following those assumptions, this will, logically, increase the production of serotonin during the morning.

Much of the most interesting research, therefore, has been to help the body use serotonin better and to keep more of it in between the brain's nerve cells in order to increase our feelings of fullness:

- One of the best examples of these attempts is dexfenfluramine—Redux. It is a "serotonin reuptake inhibitor." What that means is that dexfenfluramine keeps the nerves from picking up the serotonin from one nerve to the other. It also helps the nerves emit serotonin from themselves.
- Another method tried with drugs is to increase the sensitivity of nerve receptors to serotonin. In fact, a mechanism much like this happens when smokers quit. Nicotine in cigarettes increase the sensitivity of the nerves to serotonin, ultimately causing a decrease in appetite. When the nicotine addiction stops, then the result is another serotonin thirst that leads to eating junk food and weight gain.

According to MIT professor Richard Wurtman, "Additional ways are known by which . . . serotonin levels can be augmented." (for example, merely increasing the amount of tryptophan).[33]

5-Hydroxytryptophan

More than 700 studies have been conducted on 5-hydroxytryptophan (5-HTP) since 1990. As we've mentioned before, 5-HTP is the gateway between tryptophan and serotonin.

Unlike serotonin alone, 5-HTP can cross the blood-brain barrier. This fact makes it possible for the brain to manufacture more serotonin.

With more serotonin available, you would assume the effects of serotonin on diet and mood would also follow. And that is exactly what science has observed.

In 1992, a group of Italian scientists gave either a placebo or 5-HTP to 20 obese women for two consecutive six-week periods. During the first six weeks, the women followed no prescribed diet. In the second six weeks, they had a diet.

During both periods the women on 5-HTP lost weight. During the four-month study, consistent feelings of fullness emerged for the study's patients. In the first six weeks, the women taking 5-HTP lost about two percent of their body weight (about 5 pounds).

Then, when combined with diet, those supplementing with 5-HTP lost another three percent of their initial weight over the subsequent six weeks. In three months, on average, they lost about 15 pounds of their original weight of about 220.

Those supplementing with 5-HTP consumed significantly less carbohydrates and calories than the others in the control group getting a placebo. (One side effect in some included nausea and vomiting, but that prospect cut down with time.)

The authors of this study wrote, "These findings together with the good tolerance observed suggest that 5-HTP may be safely used to treat obesity."[34]

An earlier but similar study occurred in the late 1980s. Over five weeks of supplementing with either a placebo or 5-HTP, 19 obese women were tested. Those with 5-HTP ate considerably less than those who supplemented with only a placebo. The average weight loss for those who supplemented with 5-HTP was about three to four pounds.

The study's authors concluded, "The good tolerance suggests this substance may be safely utilized in the long-term treatment of obesity."[35]

Similarly, J.E. Blundell, a professor of biopsychology in Leeds, England, and a leading researcher in 5-HTP, said studies of 5-HTP and diet extend back at least to the mid-'80s. At least three studies, for example, showed that rats, when given 5-HTP as a supplement, were much less hungry than rats in a control group, even when those consuming 5-HTP were also given a deprived diet.[36]

5-HTP to Combat Depression

Though the human studies linking 5-HTP and the control of obesity showed little evidence of 5-HTP being connected with a change in mood, significant research seems to show that 5-HTP can help combat depression for some people.

In a 1988 study, for example, 25 depressed patients were treated with 5-HTP and the benefits of 5-HTP "was considered equal to that of traditional antidepressants."[37]

In another significant study, Dr. W. Poldinger of the Psychiatrische Universitatsklinik in Basel, Switzerland, in a double blind, multi-center, controlled study used patients diagnosed with depression. Dr. Poldinger found that after 6 weeks, both patients taking 100 mg of 5-HTP 3 times per day and those taking 150 mg of Prozac—fluvoxamine—3 times per day showed about 50 percent improvement in their depression. Those taking 5-HTP also had a better tolerance for the therapy and a lower failure rate.[38]

On the other hand, some research shows some of the more severe cases of depression may, in fact, be caused by a breakdown of the process that allows 5-HTP itself to cross into the brain.[39] This line of research also adds strong evidence to the fact that in other types of depression, 5-HTP would logically be a significant alternative to traditional therapies.

Griffonia simplicifolia

That brings us to *Griffonia simplicifolia*, a plant that grows in the savannah grasslands and coastal plains of Ghana and other countries of West Africa. It is a climber in the secondary forests and is cultivated for its many uses.

West Africans use the plant's hard wood for walking sticks and its stem and root as chewing sticks. The leaves are fed to sheep and goats to aid in reproduction. In humans, the leaves help in the healing of wounds. The leaf juice is a traditional enema and treatment for kidney ailments. A combination of stem and leaf is used to stop vomiting and is also used as an aphrodisiac.[40]

The seeds—the legumes—of *Griffonia simplicifolia* contain about 12 percent total 5-HTP. Since the West African people have used the plant for medicine and food for generations, there is strong evidence of its safe use as a long-term approach to aid in our battles for self-control against obesity.

That means griffonia, unlike Redux, is something that, thanks to its historical uses, may represent a long-term solution to weight management when included in a broad plan of lifestyle management. It accomplishes, through 5-HTP, the same result as the now-banned drug but through a different mechanism.[41]

The Tryptophan Controversy

For about 40 years following WWII, millions of doses of tryptophan were consumed by Americans to help them deal with insomnia, depression and pain. Many spoke devotedly of its benefits.

Then tragedy struck. It became what may be the worst such drug or supplement tragedy since the thalidomide scare of the 1960s. Any discussion of tryptophan and its related chemicals would be incomplete without exploring this important story.

You may have heard that tryptophan caused awful results. That would be wrong. The reality is, however, that virtually all, if not all, of the problems were caused by the manufacturer— an impurity was present in the tryptophan capsules. The story is as follows:

In 1989, people taking tryptophan supplements began to experience painful symptoms. Their joints hurt. Their mouths broke out in ulcers. They felt weak. By mid-June 1990, the United States Center for Disease Control found more than 1,500 cases of a blood allergic-type condition called Eosinophilia Myalgia Syndrome, EMS, with 31 associated deaths.

Many people began to see a connection of tryptophan and the reputation of this amino acid as a supplement suffered grievous harm before the truth came out.

Many cases were similar to that of Marilyn Rumph, who lived near Washington D.C. She took tryptophan for the successful relief—the success is important—of minor, chronic pain for about two years until, in the summer of 1989, she began to suffer strange symptoms. Her skin became swollen and reddened. Strange lesions appeared. She felt intense pain, constant fatigue and stayed in bed. She appeared before Congress two years later to complain of her condition, and she still had not healed completely. Instead, she looked forward to a life of chronic pain.[42]

Over time, officials learned that tryptophan was not, in fact, to blame. Rather, a Japanese company, Showa Denka, made a mistake in the manufacturing process, and contaminants had caused the problems.

There is on-going research about tryptophan and 5-HTP and their roles in diseases like EMS and scleroderma, a skin-hardening condition, but the results seem to indicate that it is, indeed, impurities that caused the problems.

In one of the most recent studies, the National Institutes of Health examined members of a family who became ill after taking 5-HTP. The 5-HTP used by the family contained an impurity not present in samples given to other patients. After a replacement of 5-HTP not containing this impurity, the problem resolved itself.[43]

So, how to sort all of this out? Here are some important considerations:

- Well-intentioned scientists disagree whether tryptophan and other single ingredients such as 5-HTP should be categorized as drugs or merely supplements. That debate will continue.
- The evidence increasingly seems to show that tryptophan and 5-HTP have a long history of safety. While occasional studies have shown some amount of stomach upset—notably nausea—and other minor side effects with the use of these supplements, few, if any, scientists see any long-term problems with the nutrients themselves. Indeed, it seems unlikely that something so essential and common to human life like tryptophan would be the direct cause of these diseases. At one level, it would be something like vitamin C preventing scurvy on the one hand while causing rickets on the other.

- As further evidence of the efficacy of tryptophan and its related supplements, the U.S. suffered from the EMS outbreak, while only 11 Canadians contracted the disease—an exact contrast to the thalidomide scare—and 10 of those were confirmed to have bought tryptophan inside the United States.[44]
- Because griffonia has a long history of cultivation and traditional use, that history provides strong evidence of safety and benefit.
- Of course, as with the majority of supplements, you may want to consult a physician before taking 5-HTP or even griffonia. If unusual joint pain, tissue pain or an unusual rash develops, stop taking the supplement—and consider dropping the other medications you are taking—and see a physician immediately, just as you would if you had an unusual reaction to aspirin.
- Similarly, if you take a mood-altering drug (notably MAO inhibitors) or some obesity medication, use extreme caution. There is research and experience to suggest that 5-HTP enhances the effect of those drugs. Also, its effect on pregnant women has never been studied so using it while pregnant should be avoided. A few other experiments have indicated that it may cause drowsiness—a natural conclusion since melatonin comes from it. So use caution if you must drive or use heavy machinery.[45]
- At least one author warns that large amounts of tryptophan supplementation, (and, perhaps, by implication, 5-HTP) might cause decreased fetal weights and higher fetal death rates in animals. Similarly, extra "excitability" might happen with those who consume tryptophan alone.[46]

In essence, as with all supplements and lifestyle issues, be wise and responsible following dosage recommendations, but there seems little cause for concern.

Some Final Thoughts about Obesity

Women like Phyllis and Laura no longer need to feel like failures for their seeming lack of self-control. Our bodies need serotonin, just as they need water. We don't need to feel too guilty over thirst, so we shouldn't feel too guilty over food cravings.

We might counter the thirst with long glasses of cool water, and we should counter the serotonin thirst with the right diet, high in tryptophan or 5-HTP—griffonia.

Remember, too, a well-balanced diet, high in vitamins and minerals is vital. Get plenty of fiber to keep your system running smoothly. Eat a sensible breakfast high in grains.

Exercise adequately. Cut down on the bad fats. Sleep well. Drink plenty of water. Eat five or more servings of fruits and vegetables each day. These simple suggestions are vital in improving your health and your chances of losing weight.

Along the way, appropriate supplements besides griffonia may also help. You might look at something like conjugated linoleic acid, an essential fatty acid, fat absorbers like chitosan (though not the two taken at the same time each day) or the short-term use of metabolism enhancers. All have their place.[47]

But remember the hopeful results of this West African plant, famous for its walking sticks. Women like Phyllis and Laura, who may be struggling without Redux, now have a new option, one that could work in the long term. Tests show women eat less and lose weight—up to 15 pounds in four months based on one study—simply by adding 5-HTP to the diet.

That's the active ingredient in griffonia, a natural alternative to Redux and the other obesity drugs.

Simply put, it's time to eliminate the guilt we associate with overeating. No more hunger artists. No more phone-booth-sized chairs. No more guilt over self-control.

It's as if we are merely thirsty. Let's take a drink. Griffonia provides a new answer to slake our serotonin thirst. Let's stop waiting and get on with better health today.

Endnotes

1. Wurtman & Wurtman, "Brain Serotonin, Carbohydrate-Craving, Obesity and Depression," 1995, a paper delivered at the 1995 conference of the International Study Group in Padova, Italy, published in *Recent Advances in Tryptophan Research*. Edited by Fillipini et. al., Plenum Press, New York, 1996.
2. Johannnes, L. and Carton, B., http://www.civilrights.com/fenphen.html. See also "Lean Times, Dieting Goes 'Natural' after Fen-Phen scare; Small Players get fat," *Wall Street Journal*, Sept. 29, 1997. See also www.fda.gov/cder/news/fenphenpr81597.htm.
3. Op. Cit. Wurtman.
4. Schwartz, Hillel, *Never Satisfied: A Cultural History of Diets, Fantasies and Fat*, 1986, The Free Press.
5. Ibid.
6. *Obesity and Weight Control: The Health Professional's Guide to Understanding and Treatment*, a collection of papers on obesity, edited by Frankle, Reva T.
7. Ibid.
8. *Proteins and Amino Acids in Nutrition*, edited by Melville Sahyun, Reinhold, N.Y. 1948.
9. Ibid.
10. *Academic American Encyclopedia*, 1997 edition, Groliers.
11. Ibid.
12. Ibid.
13. *Encyclopedia Britannica*, 15th edition.

14. B. Witkop, "Retro, Intro. and Perspective on Trypto-Fun," In *Kynurenine and Serotonin Pathways*, edited by Schwarcz, et. al., 1991, Plenum Press.
15. *Modern Nutrition in Health and Disease*, 6th edition, Goodhard and Shils, editors, published by Lea and Febiger, 1980.
16. *The Nutrition and Health Encyclopedia*, Tyler, D.F. & Russell, P., Van Reinhold, 1981.
17. *Nutrients Catalog*, Newstrom Harvey, McFarland, 1993.
18. Ibid. and Delhaye, S. and Landry, J., "The Tryptophan Content in Protein of Cereal Grains and Legume Seeds as a Function of Nitrogen Content, A Reappraisal of Tryptophan Score," in *Recent Advances*, #1 above.
19. Clackson, T. and Wells J.A., 1995, "A Hot Spot of Binding Energy in a Hormone-Receptor Interface," *Science* 267:383. See also Brown, R.R., "Metabolism and Biology of Tryptophan, Some Clinical Implications," in *Recent Advances*, #1 above.
20. Simon N. Young, Opening address of the ISTRY conference in 1995 in Padova, Italy, see *Recent Advances*, #1 above.
21. "Tryptophan and Epilepsy," Lunardi, et. al., in *Recent Advances*, #1 above.
22. De La Torre, J.C., "A possible role for 5-Hydroxytryptamine in drug-induced seizures." *J. Pharmacol* 22 (1970):858.
23. Milovanovic, D.D., et. al., "Plasma Tryptophan Levels in the Patients with Cervicobrachial and Lumbosacral Pain Syndromes," in *Recent Advances*, #1 above.
24. Weil-Fugazze, J., "Endogenous Kynurenine Derivatives and Pain," in *Recent Advances*, #1 above. See also interview with Lori Blackner, Spring 1998, as referenced in #41 below.
25. S. Salmon, et. al., "The Possible Role of Tryptophan in Migraine," in *Recent Advances*, #1 above.
26. Young, S.N., et. al., "The Effect of Low Brain Serotonin on Mood and Aggression in Humans," in *Recent Advances*, #1 above.
27. Heyes, M.P., et. al. "Inter-relationships between quinolinic acid, neuroactive kynurenine, neopterin and B2-microglobulin in cerebrospinal fluid and serum of HIV-1 infected patients." *J. Neuroimmunol* 40(1992):71.
28. "Serotonin: The Neurotransmitter for the 90's," *Drug Topics*. 1994, October 10:108.
29. Blundell, J.E., "Serotonin and Appetite," *Psychopharmacology*, 23, 12B,

1537-1551, 1984, Pergamon Press Ltd.
30. Lytle, LD, 1977, "Control of Eating Behavior," in Wurtman RJ, Wurtman JJ, eds. *Nutrition and the Brain*. Raven Press, New York.
31. Fanelli, et al., "Tryptophan and Secondary Anorexia," in *Recent Advances*, #1 above.
32. Wurtman, R.J. & Wurtman, J.J, "Brain Serotonin, Carbohydrate-craving, Obesity and Depression," in *Recent Advances*, #1 above.
33. Ibid.
34. Cangiano, C., et al., "Eating Behavior and Adherence to Dietary Prescriptions in Obese Adult Subjects Treated with 5-hydroxytryptophan," *Am J. Clin Nutr.* 56 (1992): 863-7.
35. Ceci F. et al., "The Effects of Oral 5-hydroxytryptophan Administration on Feeding Behavior in Obese Adult Female Subjects, *J. Neural Transm.* 76 (1989) :109-117.
36. Blundell, J.E., "Serotonin and Appetite," *Psychopharmacology*, 23 (1984): 12B, 1537-1551.
37. "L-5-Hydroxytryptophan Alone and in Combination with a Peripheral Decarboxylase Inhibitor in the Treatment of Depression," Zmilacher, K. et al., *Neuropsychobiology*, 1988; 20 (1): 28-35.
38. "A Functional-Dimensional Approach to Depression: Serotonin Deficiency as a Target Syndrome in a Comparison of 5-Hydroxytriptophan (5-HTP) and Fluvoxamine." *Psychopathology*, 24 (1991): 53-81.
39. Nolen, W.A., et al., "Treatment Strategy in Depression II. MAO Inhibitors in Depression Resistant to Cyclic Antidepressants: Two Controlled Crossover Studies with Tranylcypromine Versus L-5-Hydroxytryptophan and Nomifensine," *Acta-Psychiatr-Scand*, 1988 Dec; 78 (6): 676-83. See also, Agren, H., et al., "Low Brain Uptake of L-[11-C]5-Hydroxytrptophan in Major Depression: A Positron Emission Tomography Study on Patients and Healthy Volunteers," *Acta-Psychiatr-Scand.*, 1991, Jun; 83(6): 449-55.
40. Dwuma-Badu, D., "Constitutents of West African Medicinal Plants XVI. Griffonin and Griffonilide, Nove Constituents of Griffonia simplicifolia," *Lloydia*, 1976, Nov. Dec.; 39(6): 385-90. Also, interview with Lori Blackner of #41 below, Spring 1998.
41. Interview with Lori Blackner, scientist with Nutraceuticals Inc., Fall 1997.
42. FDA's Regulation of the Dietary Supplement L-Tryptophan: Hearing before the Human Resources and Intergovernmental Relations

Subcommittee of the Committee on Government Operations, House of Representatives, One Hundred Second Congress, first session, July 18, 1991.
43. Michelson D, et al., "An Eosinophilia-Myalgia Syndrome Related Disorder Associated with Exposure to L-5-Hydroxytryptophan," *J. Rheumatol.* 1994 Dec; 21(12): 2261-5.
44. Op. Cit. FDA hearing before Congress, 1991.
45. *Nutrition Science News*, February 1998 edition, www.nutritition-sciencesnews.com.
46. Op. Cit. McFarland.
47. *CLA: Conjugated Linoleic Acid*, Williams, L. Woodland Publishing, 1997.